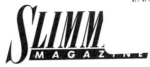

the d í'et'er's d ĭ'ctĭonar̆y

with
Warrens by Rosie

ARGUS BOOKS

dieter's dictionary

Definitions by Slimming Magazine
Readers (see page 64)

Illustrations by Rosie

Edited by Sybil Greatbatch

Designed by Carolyne Sibley

First published by Argus Books 1990
Copyright © Slimming Magazine 1990

ISBN 1 85486 038 0

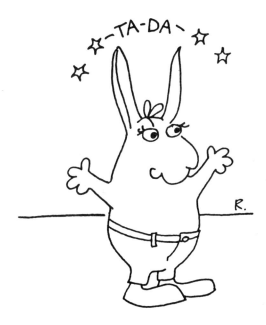

Introduction

When you are dieting, words tend to take on deeply different meanings. From the moment it first appeared in Slimming Magazine in 1986, the unique Dieter's Dictionary struck a ruefully riotous chord with readers. And they have been contributing to its continuing success ever since.

Now Dieter's Dictionary definitions are collected here to spread the fun further. And for extra amusement, the book is illustrated with another favourite Slimming regular: Rosie's popular "Warrens" cartoons. Warrens will strike a sympathetic chord with all slimmers, past and present.

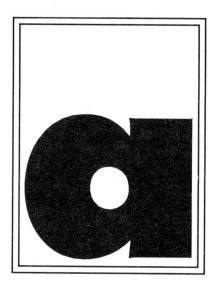

abstinence:
going without eating for 8 hours — from 11pm to 7am

acceptable weight:
what you weigh now if you were six inches taller

aerobics:
biscuits covered with bubbly milk chocolate

aerobics:
activity you will get down to when you have finished this doughnut to keep your strength up

aerobics:
sprinting to reach the cake shop just before it shuts

aerobics:
a bar of chocolate followed by two biscuits

After Eight Mints:
after eight, you might as well finish the box off

aromatherapy:
smells so good I'll feel better if I eat it all

afters:
courses that helped create your 'before' photographs

astronomical:
measurements due to fanatical interest in Galaxy, Milky Way and Mars

ambidextrous:
ability to eat with one hand whatever the other hand is doing

average portion:
roughly a quarter of what you usually eat

ambidextrous:
being able to clasp a cream doughnut in one hand while holding a fistful of peanuts in the other

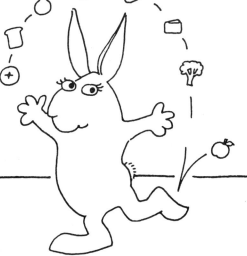

R.

ambition:
trying to slim your way from Evans to Next

appetite:
the only thing that's more ferocious than next-door's Dobermann

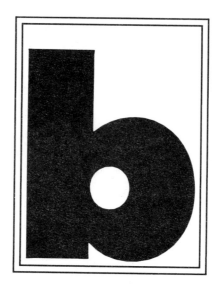

back end of a bus:
safest place to eat a Mars bar in secret

bain-marie:
washing biscuits retrieved from the bin

baked potato:
high-fibre container for four ounces of butter

baker's dozen:
biscuits that disappear while still warm from the oven

balanced eating:
a Mars bar in each hand

balanced meal:
me carrying a piled-high plate

banquet:
where the table groans
before you do

bar code:
automatically seeking the diet
drinks

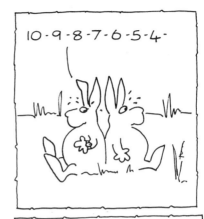

bath:
an ever-narrowing device for
getting washed in

bathroom scales:
cheater beater

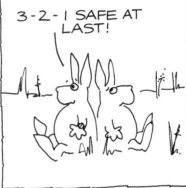

bathroom scales:
equipment which only seems
to work correctly when
one holds on to towel rail,
stands on one foot and
leans hard to the left

bedtime:
calorie allowance all eaten

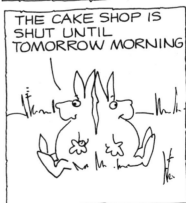

dieter's dictionary

belt:
strip of leather that shrinks in direct proportion to wearer's willpower

bigamy:
somebody who would much prefer to be little Amy

big-boned:
a person who isn't fat but looks it

bikini:
swimwear you insist is no longer in fashion

bikini:
article of clothing worn by women who never eat

bikini:
garment as inaccessible, alas, as a certain Pacific island

biscuits:
food items noteworthy because broken ones' calories don't count

bitter memory:
not had a drink for a week

black coffee:
liquid used to wash down fresh cream gateaux

blusher:
coloured powder used in attempts to discover cheekbones

body-building
exercise to re-position your bulges

body clock:
internal chronometer invariably stuck at snack-time

boob tubes:
leg-warmers for larger ladies

boring:
containing fewer than 50 calories

boss:
someone who never offers to
buy you lunch except when
you have finally decided to
diet

bottom:
something that becomes
visible when the biscuit barrel
becomes empty

box of chocolates:
offering invariably bought for
you during the first week of a
diet

BSc:
Bakes Scrumptious (small)
cakes

bunch of flowers:
offering invariably presented
when you are not on a diet
and are dying for chocolates

bus:
vehicle with stupidly narrow
seats

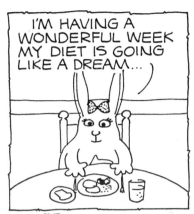

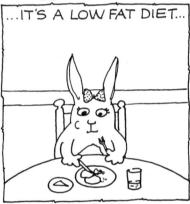

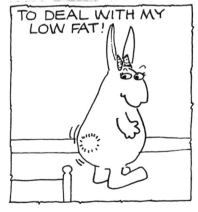

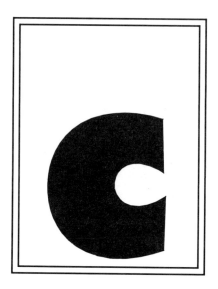

cake, cake, cake:
a gain and a gain and a gain

calorie content:
how you feel after three
gateau slices

**calorie-counted
meals:**
food which would taste fine if
served with chips

calories:
weighty substances that sink
to the bottom

Cambridge diet:
not eating anything that's
light blue

car:
a means of getting the Indian
takeaway home while still hot

carbohydrate:
a mixture of carbon, hydrogen and oxygen which trebles in mass on contact with the hips

cat flap:
the fuss which that skinny woman down the road makes when she puts on a pound

celeriac:
somebody with the heart to stick to life without cheese

celery:
low-calorie vegetable designed for dipping into high-calorie mayonnaise

cellulite:
attempted fraud by dishonest greengrocer

charmer:
fellow dieter who cuts you a large slice and a sliver for herself

Cheddar gorge:
six cheese sandwiches straight off

chopsticks:
the safest implement for eating chocolate mousse

Christmas:
dieter's two-months' break

Chubb lock:
size 18 woman stuck inside a size 14 dress

C.I.A:
Completely Insatiable Appetite

clock:
timepiece that doesn't tick fast enough between meals

clothes:
items that are guaranteed to reduce in size every time that they are hung up in the wardrobe

clotted cream:
cream produced for clots

coffee:
something to drink while you eat biscuits

colleague:
thin person who treats you to a coffee-time bun

comfort eating:
undoing your waistband before the meal

communication:
being able to talk with your mouth full

complex carbohydrates:
nutrients with a difficult-to-calculate calorie content

compromise:
eating a Mars bar with a Diet Coke

compromise:
switching to orange-flavoured chocolate

compulsive liar:
any speak-your-weight machine

concourse:
month's supply of expensive 'slimming' pills

condensed milk:
expansive calories

considerate husband:
one who says: 'Mind your fingers!' as you bolt a forbidden chocolate bar

controlled eating:
not actually chewing while sleeping

conversation:
an excuse to talk about food

conveyor belt:
strip of leather carrying the message that it's much too tight

correct weight:
the reading on your scale if you were three inches taller

counter intelligence:
deciding not to buy the Mars bar after all

cowl neck:
somewhere to store your chins

cravat:
fashion accessory which covers a multitude of chins

cream crackers:
dieters driven mad with desire for Devonshire teas

crumbs of comfort:
everybody knows that broken biscuits don't count

cupboard love:
devouring all cakes, biscuits and sweets in sight so that your children will grow up slim

cupboard love:
I love my food cupboard and everything in it

cutting out:
snipping size label from clothes

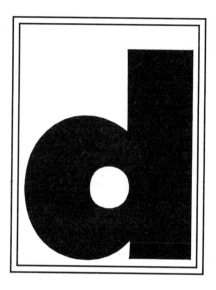

daily dozen:
five doughnuts, four Kit Kats, two plates of chips and a chunk of Cheddar

daily dozen:
chocolate digestives

daily exercise:
taking sweet wrappers to the litter bin in the park before husband gets home

dangerous additive:
extra spoonful after weighing out your portion

day-dreaming:
being cast away on a dessert island

deception:
setting bathroom scales back 2st in case anyone comes in while you're weighing

deck-chair:
person-trap found on open ground

dedication:
spending an hour and a half contriving a recipe for low-calorie mince pies

defeat:
what I used to be able to see before debulge

defrosting freezer:
task which involves eating one whole Black Forest Gateau and two dozen sausage rolls

de-icer:
friend who quietly cuts you a topless slice of Christmas cake

deposit account:
confessing to friends how you put it all on

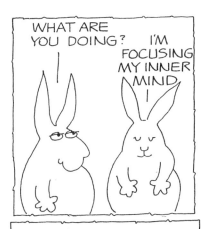

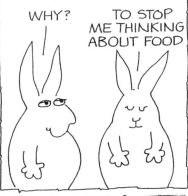

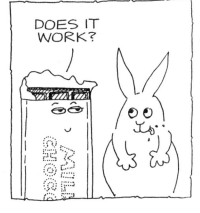

dieter's dictionary

depression:
no longer being wolf-whistled when passing a building site

depression:
finding the supermarket has closed early

deprivation:
result of supermarket closing early

desk drawer:
compartment designed to hold crisps and biscuits

desperation:
eating the dog's choc drops

desperation:
cutting toenails before stepping on scales

detente:
on outsize dress from Paris

diatonic:
morale-booster of losing two pounds

diatribe:
whole family of slimmers

diatribe:
weight loss plan for entire family

diet scale:
eater meter

dipstick:
zip that, once down, won't do up again

distinguished guest:
the fattest person at a party

doctor:
person who believes you to be incredibly fit because you steer clear in case he mentions your weight

Doomsday Book:
daily record of what you've eaten

double feature:
extra chin due to constant over-snacking in cinemas

doughnut:
low-calorie cake due to its entirely non-fattening centre

dream holiday:
being accidentally locked inside a chocolate factory for at least a week

dressing table:
where you lie to zip up your jeans

duty free:
solitary consumption of a whole box of chocolates — no sharing necessary!

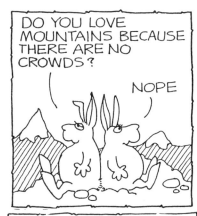

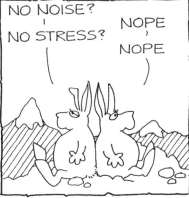

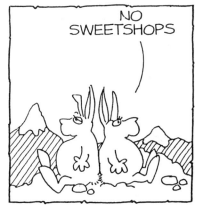

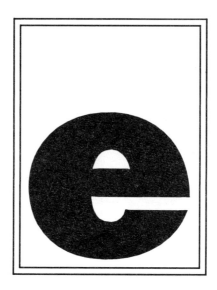

Easter egg:
a gift so bad for the children that you have to eat it yourself

eating for two:
finishing husband's pudding because he's had quite enough

economy:
buying Mars bars in packs of three

ecstasy:
falling into a great vat of chocolate and having to eat your way out

elevenses:
snack eaten between tenses and twelveses

eloquent:
someone able to talk for 20 minutes about the goodness contained in chocolate

empty calories:
the kind that fill you up the best

entente cordiale:
sugary drink for fat campers

Eve:
only woman ever really tempted by an apple

exercise:
the-er-size you used to be

exercise bike:
a handy piece of equipment on which to hang leotards

eXtra Large:
dress size you can judge even without looking at the label

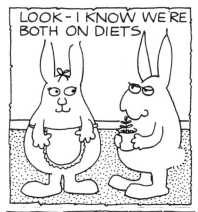

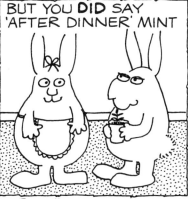

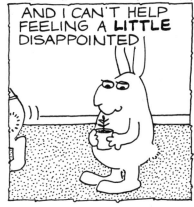

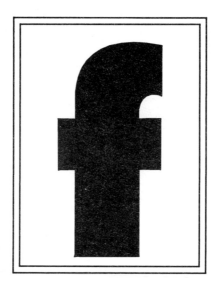

facial sauna:
head hung over a steaming
mug of hot chocolate

fast:
the most satisfying way to get
to the fridge

fad:
Failed Another Diet

fat:
substance which looks more
on than off

family-size pack:
just enough for you

fat (pound of):
represents 3,500 calories
when you try to lose it but only
350 when it gains on you

fat friend:
someone who makes you look thinner more efficiently than all the vertical stripes in the world

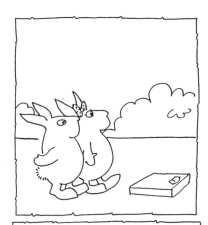

fatigue:
tiredness at being overweight

fatted calf:
located between the fatted knee and fatted ankle

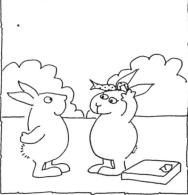

fatty tissue:
sneeze of someone who's overweight

fat unit:
me!

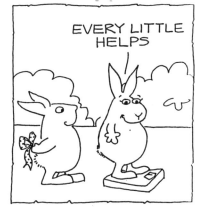

fat units:
fitted-kitchen cupboards full of baddies

faulty scales:
lying in weight

fed up:
what one is once one has

festive fare:
unfairly fattening

fiction:
I've lost all craving for chocolate

filofax, (phyllofax):
awful truth about calorie content of a certain continental pastry

five-course meal:
pre-dinner nibbles; starter; main course; dessert; left-overs

flan:
next to flab in the dictionary

flattering:
any shade that's black

fluid retention:
two bottles of gin secreted in the sideboard

food mountain:
me

foodstuff:
anything worth a really big binge

form-filling:
alternative description for particularly delicious high-calorie foods

freezing glance:
quick check to see that there are still ample stocks of Cornettos

French francs:
outspoken comments on your size when you sunbathe on the Cote d'Azur

fridge:
device used in summer to prevent chocolate from melting

frigidity:
cold fear of the consequences of opening refrigerator

fruit:
raw filling for rich pastry pies

frustration:
size tens on the washing-line next door

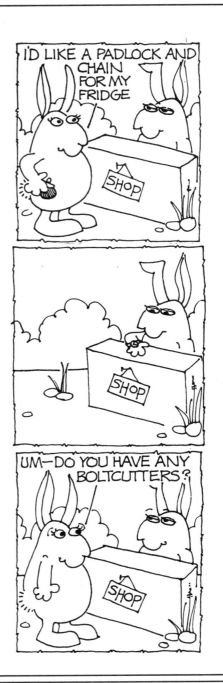

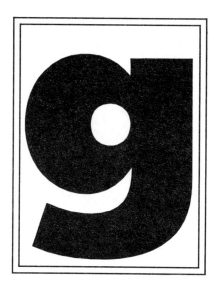

garage:
place to keep emergency store of biscuits, chocolates and crisps

garden shed:
back-yard skipping-rope sessions

G.C.S.E:
Gooey Cream Slice/Eclair

gear lever:
favourite too-tight dress that finally forces you to diet

generosity:
offering to eat your friend's second cream cake so that she won't get fat

gentle hint:
you make Luciano Pavarotti look like an anorexic flea

German marks:
bruises sustained when fighting over the last apple strudel

going for the burn:
eating the crunchy black bits at the bottom of the chip bag

going vegetarian:
eating fruit-and-nut chocolate instead

Good Friday:
dieting day usually preceding Bad Saturday, Sunday and Monday

great divide (the):
zippy gap at the top of your jeans

great time:
there was loads to eat

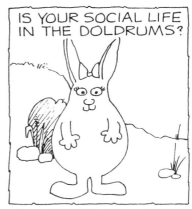

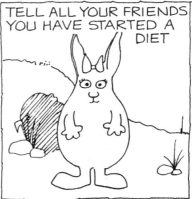

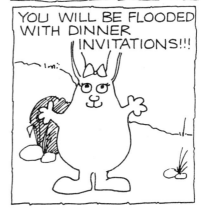

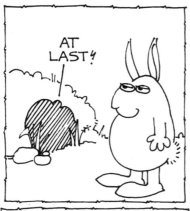

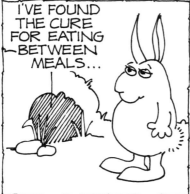

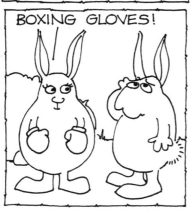

green consumer:
someone who sincerely
believes water biscuits to be
calorie-free

greenpeace:
honestly trying to come to
terms with cabbage

green salad:
a pretty accompaniment for
pork pies

grill:
what a dieter uses as an
emergency defroster for
cheesecake

gruyere:
cheese that isn't holely
fattening

guilty conscience:
a condition marginally less
painful than hunger

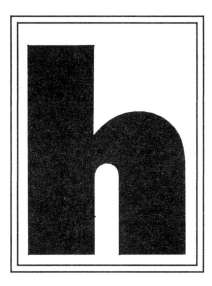

half-the-fat spread:
twice as much on the bread

handbag:
a kind of constant picnic basket

handful:
what the two peanuts you decided to nibble turn into

hangover:
the roll of fat just above one's firm-control girdle

happiness:
going into a changing-room with dresses in two sizes and finding that the smaller one fits

happy hour:
period of blissful ignorance before stepping on scales

dieter's dictionary

heavy duty:
obligation to eat every mouthful of hugely high-calorie meal that your mother has made for you

high fibre:
tall person wearing inexpensive wig

high fibre:
bran breakfast cereal stored at top of kitchen cupboard in order to leave room for biscuits on a more accessible shelf

historical knowledge:
the Battle Of The Bulge, Custard's Last Stand, The Duke of Beef Wellington, The Grand Old Duke of Yorkshire Pudding, Garibaldi The Biscuit Man

hope:
buying a Mars bar along with a diet cola

horse sense:
refusing a pony ride at the fair

hot cross bun:
bakery item consumed after long and losing struggle to zip up jeans

humiliation:
'Have you got this in a larger size, please?'

husband:
specimen of animal species with unique ability to eat only half a Mars bar

hydrotherapy:
I'll feel better if someone hides it

hypoglycaemia:
dangerous drop in blood sugar level occurring after three hours' deprivation of chocolate-coated raisins; preventable

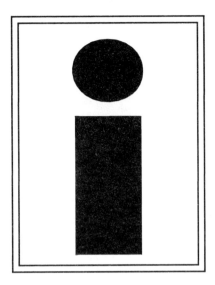

ideal husband:
one who revels in soft rotundity

ideal weight chart:
information invoking desire to be a 6-ft-4 man

I mustn't
I will but tempt me some more first, please

indignation:
emotion felt when scales read the same after removal of earrings, makeup and going to the loo

insinuate:
naughty nibble during strict dieting

intellectual:
sings 'O Sole Mio' to the tune of 'Just One Cornetto'

I shouldn't:
try and stop me

interface:
where the food goes

interfering:
adjective for well-meaning woman next door who gives you gift tokens from the local hardware store at Christmas because 'I didn't think someone like you would want anything frivolous such as makeup'

international trade:
importing Swiss chocolate

Italian lire:
cheeky looks from Romans who fancy fat women

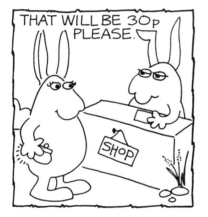

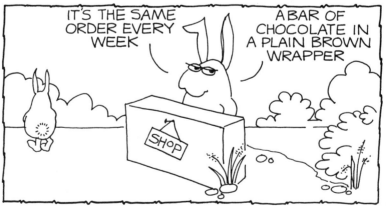

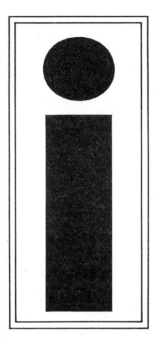

jeans:
thank goodness, that explains why they don't fit me

jeans:
pair of denim trousers guaranteed to shrink at least two sizes a year

jeans:
large enough, alas, to be Jim's

jelly mould:
corset

jogging:
reaching the sweetshop slightly faster than if one had walked there

jolly:
what everyone swears you used to be before you lost weight, though you feel much happier now

dieter's dictionary

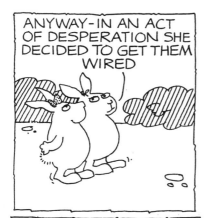

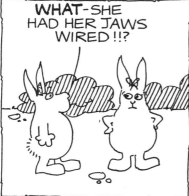

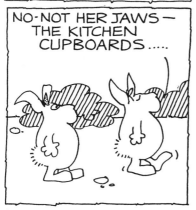

joystick:
the support in the centre of candyfloss

justice:
when your I-can-eat-anything best friend finally puts on a considerable amount of weight

justify:
saying 'it won't make much difference if I just eat this one cream cake,' etc

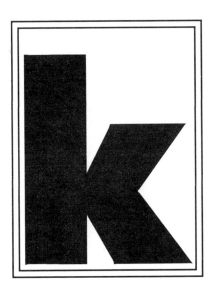

kitchen scale:
useful for weighing out
chocolate-cake ingredients

Krepton Factor:
why those mysterious extra
pounds appeared

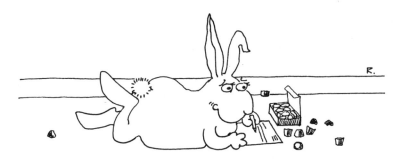

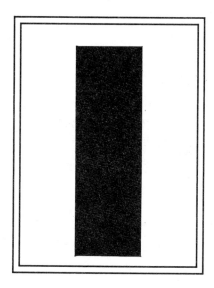

lack of incentive:
I've bought a skirt with an
elasticated waist

lateral thinking:
lying in bed yearning for
Yorkie Bars

Lady Bountiful:
somebody bulging because of
a certain chocolate-bar brand

leotard:
stretchy garment that needs
to be

late-night viewing:
a wee-small-hours peep into
the pantry

light eaters:
when it's light, they eat

liposuction:
technique used by advanced gourmands on particularly long pieces of buttery spaghetti

London:
place where food shops stay open all night

longest day:
when you've consumed your total calorie allowance by noon

low-cal:
you can eat twice as much before you put on weight

low-calorie:
bar of chocolate eaten while dusting under the bed

low-calorie:
eating the biscuit you dropped on the floor

low-fat:
adipose deposits below the waistline

low-fat:
puffy ankles

low-fat spread:
my bottom's getting bigger

low-fat spread:
dinner on the floor due to collapse of last dining-chair

low-fat spread:
my bottom in jeans

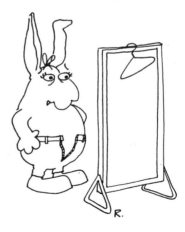

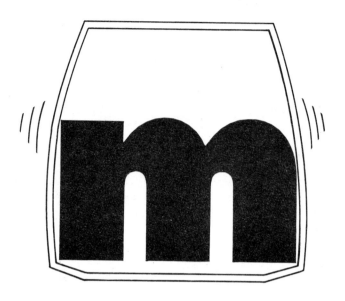

manicure:
something to have if the rest of you is Too Awful to do anything with

marathon training:
jogging in an attempt to make up for recently eaten chocolate bar

market forces:
the lady at the cake stall is so persuasive

marriage:
a couple, one of whom is on a diet

marsupial:
one always able to carry a secret Mars bar

maturity:
more waist, less speed

maximum:
overweight mother

McDonald's shake:
meeting your Slimming Magazine Club Group Leader on the way out

mealtime:
eating off a plate instead of straight from the packet

meal times:
set periods that interrupt snacking

meditation:
meaningful moments spent thinking about Mars bars

metabolic rate:
always lower than your rate of inflation

metabolism:
body mechanism naturally set to burn up at least 1,000 calories fewer daily than you have consumed

Michelin Guide:
where to get a rather expensive spare tyre

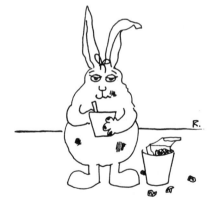

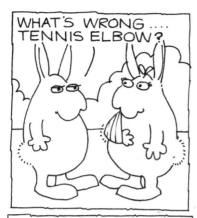

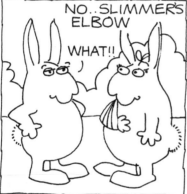

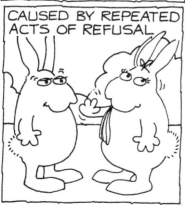

microwave:
an invention which makes two
minutes seem like a lifetime

**middle-aged
spread:**
unconquered puppy fat

mint lumps:
due to over-indulgence in
After Eights

misconception:
blaming chocolate cravings
on what turns out to be
another phantom pregnancy

misjudgment:
leaving the bread knife near
the fruit cake

moderation:
half now, half later

moral fibre:
eating All-Bran in church

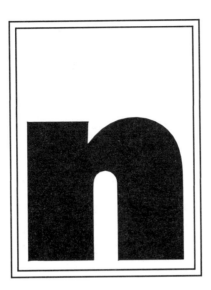

narrow escape:
the dog reaching the plate of biscuits a second before you do

no artificial colourings:
this product contains preservatives and artificial flavourings

no artificial flavourings:
contains preservatives and artificial colourings

no preservatives:
guaranteed to go off as soon as opened

no thanks:
a phrase which a slimmer can't use because it hurts other people's feelings

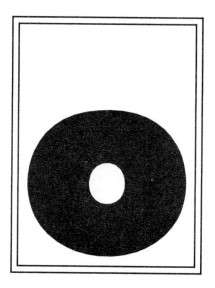

one-size tights:
the size is never yours

one-size tights:
you're the one size they are
not designed to fit

optimism:
hoping that low-cal
doughnuts will shortly be
invented

optimist:
somebody who buys a
month's allowance of treats
in one go

optimist:
looking under the brown
paper in a chocolate box to
see if there's a third layer

optimum:
a mother who firmly believes
that this diet will work

O.S:
Orange Squash

ounce:
cheese you place on the scales
after biting off a carefully
calculated chunk

over the top:
when your bra decides that
you should slim

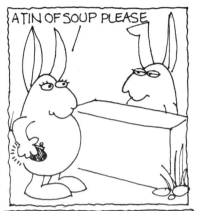

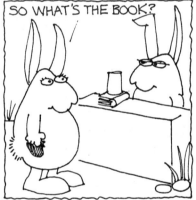

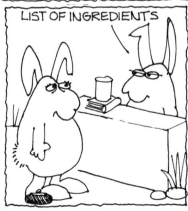

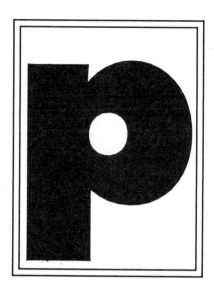

packed lunch:
greedily crammed carrier bag

perfect fit:
the button doesn't actually
burst when you breathe

pantry:
household area calling for
constant tidying

pie in the sky:
only safe place for it

piggy bank:
cash reserved for chocolate,
crisps, etc

peanuts:
what you used to think their
calorie content was!

pig ignorant:
no idea of the calories in a pork chop

pleasantly plump:
used by slim people as a kindly compliment (see also: bonny, comely and 'You're looking well')

P.M.T:
Permanently Meal Time

P.M.T:
Post-Meal Trauma or realization that you've just eaten 4,000 calories

politeness:
accepting chocolate in order not to offend

pot luck:
finally finding a girdle that fits

pregnancy:
sigh of relief for nine months

press-ups:
loose-bottomed cake tins

public humiliation:
a snapped knicker elastic and consequent collapse while passing a building site and realizing not one labourer has batted an eyelid

puppy fat:
substance that drips off the end of a hot-dog

puppy fat:
excuse for not starting a diet till you're 30

puppy fat:
what Mother said 'would simply vanish' — in 1977

puppy fat:
caused by eating your poodle's choccy-drops in a very bad moment

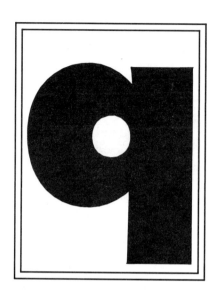

quilt:
bed cover that must have shrunk

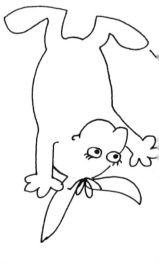

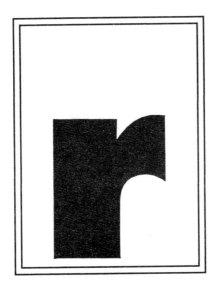

reduction:
always most noticeable in the body area where you least want to lose weight

regular exercise:
frequent trips to the refrigerator; not to be confused with violent exercise (running to the refrigerator)

reincarnation:
returning to live another life as a tin of milk

rhinestone:
what you gain on a German holiday

ribs:
succulent sticks of meat served with rich sauce

dieter's dictionary

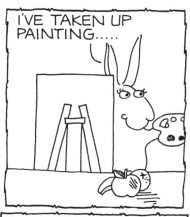

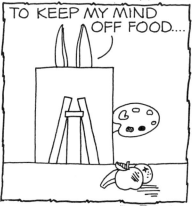

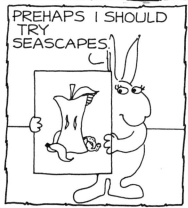

rock 'n' roll:
how we danced then, how we walk now

roses:
flowers with soft and hard centres

R.S.P.B:
Regretting a Splurge of Peanut Butter

R.S.P.C.A:
Reasonable Success in Preventing Chocolate Abuse

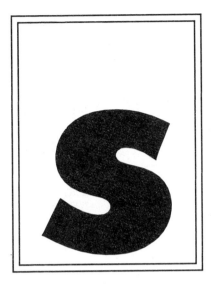

saccharin:
little tablets you drop in the liquid you drink with thickly buttered toast

salad:
food that tastes terrific when garnished by a crusty buttered roll and large chunk of cheese

saturated fat:
what sticks out beyond the limits of an umbrella

scales:
what fall from your eyes when you add up the calories you really ate today

scarf:
accessory covering a multitude of chins

seafood:
all you need to do to make you eat it

second helpings:
the first helping of food before the third

secret service:
friend who smuggles in forbidden food during your health-farm stay

seismology:
study of girthquakes

self-confidence:
passing a full-length mirror and not feeling forced to look

self-control:
leaving one Malteser in the box

self-control:
throwing away the crisp bag without ripping it open to get the bits out of the corners

self-deception:
going into a chip shop in order to ask the way

self-deception:
buying chocolate biscuits for one's husband to eat

set meal:
an occasion for eating everything included in the price

shift dress:
its tightness shocks you into slimming

shortcake:
eclair eaten in five seconds flat

shorts:
very small alcoholic drinks

shouldn't:
but I will, and what's more, I'll put the blame on you!

shower:
good reason for sheltering in a sweet shop

shrink:
what happens to your clothes in the wash, while everybody else's stay the same size

size 12:
they no longer make it like they used to

skill:
ability to steer supermarket trolley down confectionery aisle with eyes closed

skimmed milk:
something which makes a bowlful of muesli slimming

skimmed milk:
Gold or Silver Top after its cream has been carefully removed to pour over one's low-calorie fruit salad

skin-tight:
last year's baggy clothes

skipping:
giving exercise a miss again

skipping:
missing breakfast but then eating double portions at lunchtime

sleeping:
something done outside the hours of eating

slim into it:
keep for a year, then throw away

slimline tonic:
a liquid that makes gin low-calorie

slimline tonic:
wolf whistle

slimming club:
a place where members tell each other how bad they've been all week, and then tell the group leader how good they've been

slimming club:
meeting place where one goes before celebrating the weekly weight loss with a slap-up meal

Slimming Magazine Club leader:
a person who likes to see less of you each week

slimming products:
things to eat more of

smalls:
what I wish mine were

Smarties:
dieters who refuse little chocolate sweets

smarty-pants:
short gasps of delight on discovering chocolate buttons that your child has mislaid

smugness:
emotion dieters feel when refusing a piece of cake twice before eating it

snack:
something you eat while cooking the day's main meal

sneaky:
eating day's main meal after going to the slimming club

soap dish:
absurdly slender star of Dallas, Dynasty, etc.

soap dish:
large snack for daily consumption while watching Neighbours

software:
satin undies that you've promised yourself when you reach target weight

spare tyre:
something that a dieter must learn to change for herself

spooning:
pigging-out with your boyfriend

sports centre:
where thin people go to keep trim

spring-cleaning:
discovering new hiding-places for sneaky snacks

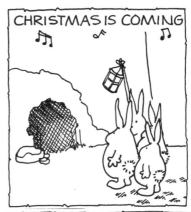

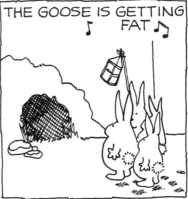

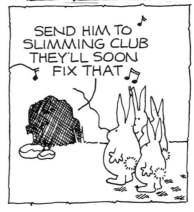

dieter's dictionary

square meal:
too many make you round

square meal:
stack of six Kit Kats

stale cake:
rumoured to be useful for
trifles but an item not known
to dieters

starter:
the beginning of the end of
your diet

stretch jeans:
garments truly suitable only
for people who don't stretch
them

sugar lump:
owner of an especially
sweet tooth

suitcase:
container for clothes that are
two sizes too small

summer dresses:
garments which shrink during
winter storage

superstition:
one more spoonful for luck

swimming pool:
a place where slim people go
to show off

syllabub:
a plan of education for the
overweight

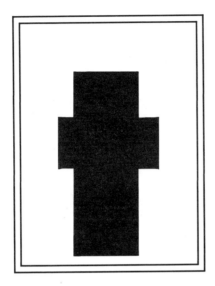

tact:
I love voluptuous women

take-aways:
things that add instead of
subtracting

tape worm:
somebody who wriggles away
from any contact with a
tape measure

tartare sauce:
saying goodbye to
high-calorie dressings

throat pastille:
something to get excited
about when all the chocolates
have gone

to diet:
verb always used in the future
tense

dieter's dictionary

tone:
sound which your muscles haven't heard of

trepidation:
emotion felt when you have put only one foot on the scales

tuna in brine:
ditty sung by slim Italian sailors

Turkey:
where delight comes from

Turkish delight:
the rumour that they adore fat women in Ankara

TV commercial:
30-second reminder of food you've spent all day trying to forget

twenty-four hour garage:
round-the-clock chocolate supply

tyre pressure:
abdominal distress after four helpings of chips

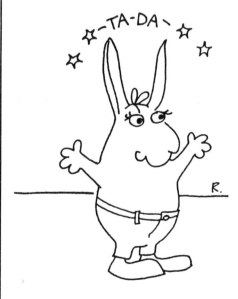

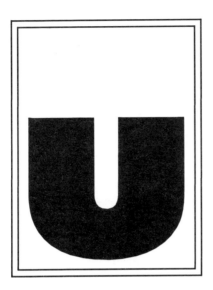

unargument-ative:

when people no longer exclaim: 'But you don't need to diet'

unavoidable:

a delicatessen 20 minutes' walk out of your way

underwire:

lifts and separates the parts you never know you had to lift and separate

unhealthy:

what thin people call you when you are fat and fat people call you when you are thin

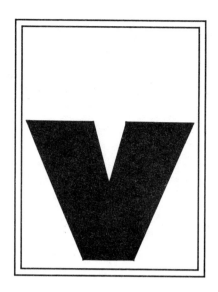

vacuum cleaner:
device to remove the evidence

V.H.F:
Very Hungry Feeling

V.A.T:
Very Active Teeth

virtuous:
a feeling you get from
refusing a fourth biscuit

V.D.U:
very dreary underwear

V.L.C.D:
Very Little Chewing Done

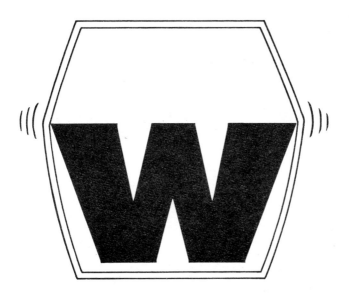

wardrobe:
a place for storing clothes which are going to fit next summer

waste not:
gain more

water polo:
eating peppermints in the bath

weigh-in:
cue for way out

weight lifting:
heaving out of one's favourite chair

well:
how people say you look when they really mean fat

dieter's dictionary

well balanced:
a small black coffee to go with a large cream cake

well-built
you're the size of a house

well-built
somebody the size of a block of flats

wholefood:
food that can be eaten in one mouthful, eg. petit fours

wholefoods:
entire fruitcakes

wholemeal:
what a slimmer can sometimes feel she never had

willpower:
a quality wasted on those who don't need it

willpower:
eating one peanut

willpower:
resisting temptation until nobody's looking

wine:
sound made when, having drunk one's calorie-counted glassful, there's some left in the bottle

wolf whistle:
hearing that the diet is working

wolf whistle:
noises you sometimes hear when driving a car, which suddenly cease when you unfold yourself out of it

wok:
regular long one with dog used as stay-slim measure by Chinese

work-out:

a programme of chewing exercises on something of a resistance consistency, preferably a Mars bar

work-out:

strenuous calorie calculations necessary for somehow cramming cream cakes into a daily 1,000 calories

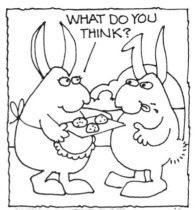

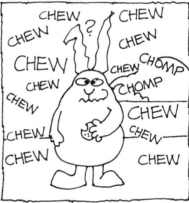

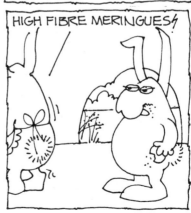

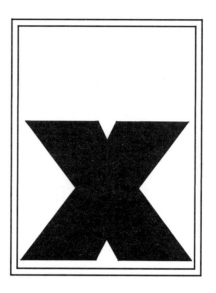

Xmas pudding:
non-Slimming reader on
Twelfth Night

X-ray:
the only photo I ever look
thin in

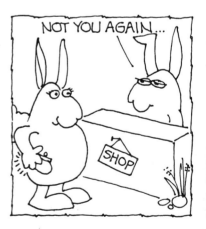

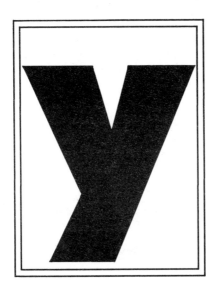

yellow pages:
reference device for locating
the nearest chip shop

yippy:
dieter who's reached target
weight

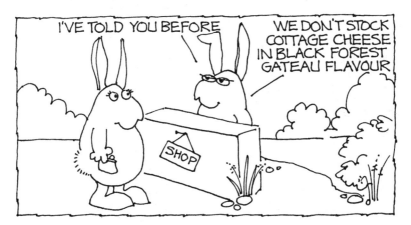

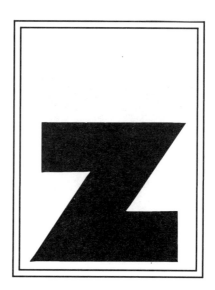

zebra:
comes after C-bra and D-bra

zen:
the contemplation of beautiful cream gateaux

zenith:
heaviest weight ever

zero hour:
time diet begins

zig-zag course:
crossing the road to avoid the baker...the sweet shop... the burger bar...etc

zip:
what will only go up when you go down

zoo:
the only safe place to go at feeding time

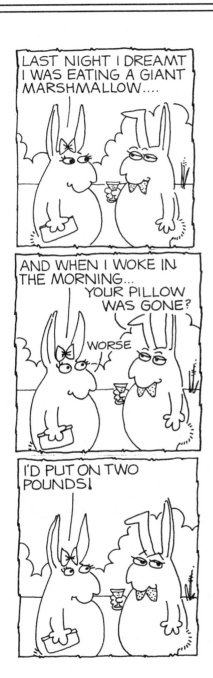

dieter's dictionary

We would like to thank the following readers who have contributed to this book with their definitions:

a M. Ackroyd; Ruth Anson; Janice Avery; Mike Ashton; L. G. Allen, Janet Ashenden;

b Lynne Blackett; E. Brock; Sarah Budd; Jean Barry; Karen Blampied; Kim Baker; Martin Barnett; J. L. Brampton-Ward; Catherine Brown; J. Bougourd; M. Bannon; Gillian Banks; Mary Brooks; R. Bennett; Melanie Bingham; A. R. Brown;

c Dr O. E. Crawshaw; P. W. Collyer; J. Cree; Alison Corfield; C. Cheyne; K. Collier; Francesca Cochonneaud; Caroline Campion; Anna Chatt Collins; Yvonne Carlile; Mary Coyne; J. Chamberlain; E. Cowdy; Janet Cowper; Linda Clarke; Marion Collins; N. Coleman; J. Cooper;

d C. A. Davis; Lynn Dearn; H. J. Dinnage; Eddy Delsasso; Joanna Dora; Jean Down; Jane Dickens; Jacqueline Donn; S. Doyley;

e Gillian Eardley; L. Edmondson; E. Edmiston;

f Margrit Forrester; Carol Fryer; D. Francis;

g Clare Giddings; M. K. Goddard; A. Gaughran; Joanna Grant; C. Gordon; Val Greaves; J. D. Goatcher; Wendy Gunneel; E. Gayle; J. Gilham;

h N. Humphreys; Diane Hutton; Sandra Haysom; Edna Harvey; C. Harding; A. G. Holmes; P. Hudson; Ann Howe; Denise Hains; Christine Hull; Sian Humphrey;

i Eve Jamieson; N. S. Jeffries; Dawn Jackson;

k D. J. Kirkpatrick; Cathy Kouvala; Linda Kettle; Jayne Kelly; Tracey Knight;

l Maura Lynch; Christine Lawrence; C. C. Lucas; Shirley Lever; D. Lee; A. Lazarus; Amanda Lee;

m Marie Middleton; Pat Mason; Jan Murray; Ann Martin; June Moore; Ann Moriaty; Karen Mares; J. McGivering; Patricia Maloney; B. Morris; Cynthia McGuigan; Jenny Modiste; Sandra Midgley; Alison Marsden; Maureen Melville;

n June Newman;

p Wendy Potts; K. Parbridge; Marion Peters; A. Palmer; R. Pearson; Vicky Penn; H. Pugh; E. Pipe; C. R. Prescot;

r K. Rowley; A. Rayment; Louise Reynolds;

s Pat Small; Ann Eleanor Spencer; A. Stewart; Susan Shaw; Freda Sumner; Julie Salt; C. Sabourin; N. Salter; J. Spurr; E. Smith;

t T. Thythal; Karen Tremeer; Fiona Teasdale; R. Thompson; Nicola Twist; Christine Thompson; Angie Tillyer;

v Jacqueline Vjesta;

w J. Wilson; Joyce Watts; W. Walker; Jan Wood; Jane Ward; J. Wilmore; A. Wallace; Wendy Worvielle; Liz Williams; J. L. Whiterod; B. Warden; Alison Worgan; P. Wood.